To Dear Buddy from one dog lover to another!

Love always,
Jane
xoxox

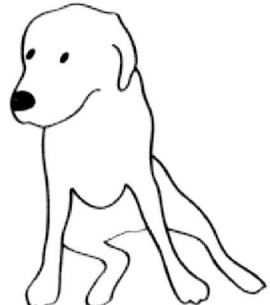

Hello.

Copyright 2011 Jane Alkon
©Mr. Boy Books, div. Jane Alkon, LLC

All Rights Reserved. Published September, 2011.

Published by Mr. Boy Books
Printed in the United States of America.

http://mrboybooks.com (http://mrboybooks.com)
MR. BOY™. THE REMARKABLE MR. BOY™. Mr. Boy™, Mr. Boy Books™ and mrboybooks.com™ are trademarks of Jane Alkon, LLC

No part of this publication may be reproduced, stored in a retrieval system, or transmitted in any form or by any means, electronic, mechanical, photocopying, recording, or otherwise without the prior written consent of the author.

Images and text contained within this publication are original and for the sole and exclusive use of Jane Alkon, LLC.

Edited by Matthew M. Jylkka

©Cover Design by Matthew M. Jylkka and Jane Alkon

©Artwork and Logo created by Matthew M. Jylkka

Library of Congress Control Number: 2011911425
ISBN 978-0-578-08807-5

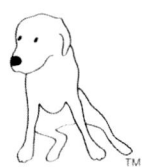

THE REMARKABLE MR. BOY

JANE ALKON

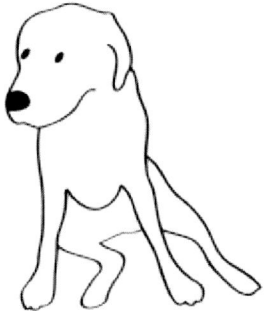

With tremendous gratitude, my thanks to
my veterinarian and friend, Dr. Heidi Mier.
Heidi has always provided incredible care
for my dogs and continues to give me
enthusiastic support in all of my
pet therapy pursuits.

Enormous thanks to Anne Hage, the Director
of the Huntington Woods Public Library.
Anne continues to extend a welcoming
hand in allowing me to bring creativity
and fun to the Library.

My love and gratitude
to my incredible family who unfailingly
encourage me in everything I do.

And finally, to my dear dog, Andy.
Always accepting, always loving,
you have opened my heart and shown
me how to share your unconditional
love with others.

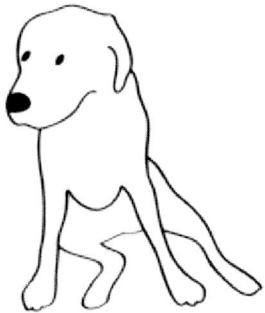

In the most unselfish and unspoiled way, dogs devote their lives to giving companionship and love.

They know of no other way to live.

Dogs never stop teaching us what is important.

Jane Alkon

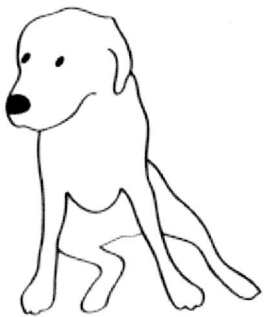

Table of Contents

Prologue	13
Just the Right Fit	16
All About Andy	20
The Road to Pet Therapy	25
Andy Visits the Hospital	31
Keisha and Andy in The Space Room	55
Saturday Mornings	61
The Ho-Hum ER	65
About Harold	68
The Library Dog is Mr. Boy	72
The Familiar Comfort of a Dog	76
Making Me Laugh	81
The Love of a Dog	84
Our Therapy Dogs	87

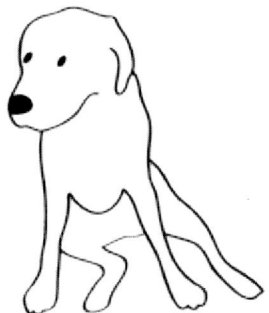

Prologue

Memories are so funny. They reveal themselves at unexpected moments and have the ability to take you back, as if time has stood still.

As my life continues to move forward, I have the love and affection of yet another dog just inches away from me. It does amaze me that at whatever stage of my life with whatever dog has provided that comfort for me, each one has had the innate ability to be the most loyal and loving companion. My four-legged friend showering me with love and adoration. In the most unequal trade, all that any of my dogs have ever demanded was to have their minimal needs met.

My dog, Andy, is an interactive bone chewer. Unlike many dogs that find a favorite bone and settle on the floor to chew away, Andy likes to have his giant nylon bone held as he chews. He often selects a favorite bone from the toy bucket, brings it over to me and I oblige him willingly. It is a true test of my own strength as I hold onto this slimy jagged nylon toy under the enormous power of his jaws.

As he chews and grinds in the natural way that dogs do, I marvel at how special he is to me. I pet his head, twirl his soft ears and tell Andy that he has unknowingly taken on the huge responsibility of being my confidant, my friend, my constant and loving companion.

I've been lucky three times so far. Each one of my incredible dogs has carried that enormous responsibility with such ease.

Even when their own lives were compromised and difficult and they were facing their final moments, *still* they had embraced their task.

I am astonished at what remarkable animals dogs really are.

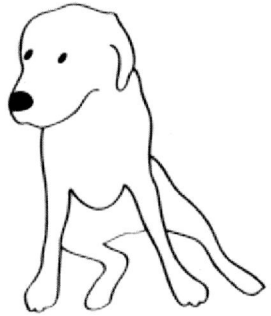

Just the Right Fit

I have always wanted a dog that followed me everywhere. Moved when I moved, watched me, hung out next to me. A dog that was a completely solid companion in every sense of the word.

Not all dogs are like that. My two female Labs were loving and adoring, but they were the ones who decided how much companionship was enough. When they had had enough of me, they were content to just have me generally within their sight. They had no need to follow every move I made.

When I thought about getting a male dog, I consulted everyone I knew who owned one. Never having had a male dog, the only thing I knew that was enormously different, aside from the obvious gender stuff, was that boy dogs lifted their legs. Ick. I didn't like that at all. It never seemed very neat or tidy to me, and certainly not very "private."

Without exception, every male dog owner assured me that I would *love* having a male dog. Unlike females, males were always cuddly and affectionate. Unlike females, males would always seek out my companionship and shadow me at every opportunity. And unlike females, males had more consistent temperaments and were more predictable, gentler dogs. From all indications, it seemed like a male dog was exactly what I was looking for.

Regardless of gender, a little puppy is a fabulous

fluff of fur. Boy or girl, you can barely resist scooping up this sweet dog and holding it closely. Cuddling is a big component in enjoying the new puppy relationship.

My dog, Andy, has always adored being held. As a nineteen pound eight-week-old puppy, it was completely luscious. With his loose skin and floppy body, it was certainly a feat to master. At thirty-five pounds, holding him was definitely a little more difficult. I figured out a way, as there was still something so delicious about holding this big bundle of love.

At almost eighty-pounds, well, that's nearly impossible. Rather than my doing most of the holding, Andy perches. Sidling next to me on the couch, Andy pivots his body around so his back is next to me. Bracing myself for his next move, he reclines, exposing his stomach and chest so I can cradle him like a giant baby. He lets his head flop and remains completely relaxed in this cradled position.

Although his heaviness is obvious, I do secretly love that he can fall asleep in this weird position with his huge body draped over me. It is one of the big pluses in having an eighty-pound lap dog.

I will admit that it is sometimes annoying that Andy cuddles so closely. I wince from the piercing jabs of his pointy elbows and am covered with his fur. I regularly find round bruises on my arms and legs that suspiciously match the size of the pads on his thick paws.

Despite all of that, as he snores away, I have little doubt that this companion was made exactly for me. Years in the making, perhaps, but, out of all of the dogs out there, Andy continues to be the exact right fit.

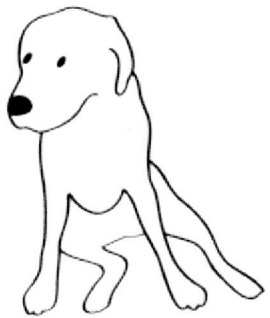

All About Andy

Dog people do not think it's strange to share your bagel with your dog. Or, give your dog half of your apple or drive your dog, in your pajamas, to the nearest drive-thru to buy a vanilla ice cream cone.

If you're a dog person, it's understood that your dog is a member of the family. On a daily basis, you talk to your dog conversationally and ask his opinion as if you actually expect an answer.

My dog, Andy, is three years old. Nicknamed "Mr. Boy," he's a purebred yellow Labrador retriever and tips the scales at eighty-pounds. He's not what you would call delicate or stealthy. He is solid though. A great big solid Labrador retriever block.

He's a bounder, running heartily toward me when I call him. Unable to get any traction, he skids across the floor and uses the closest wall as his braking system.

He is completely unaware of his size. Andy naturally squeezes into the smallest space left on the couch. He makes himself comfy as he curls into a ball on a chair, unaware his body hangs over the seat.

Andy is a nestler, a big-time cuddler and an enormous licker with dark, soulful eyes that are more expressive than you can imagine.

When you bring a dog home, you have an idea of what you think the dog's role will be. Many people simply want a family pet, adding that fun and excitement that a dog can so easily add. For others, dogs are companions offering comfort after the loss of a loved one. Still others, dogs are hunting companions or watchdogs. The list goes on and on.

Andy came into my life after my beloved dog, Bailey, passed away. For the two months I was without a dog, the quiet in the house was deafening. Every dog owner who has experienced that loss immediately notices the atmosphere in the house has changed. There was no energy, no excitement. It was simply a place for me to keep my stuff and sleep. As a consummate dog person, life without a dog was scattered, lonely and unorganized.

Andy came home with me on a bitter cold Saturday, in January 2008. From the moment I carried him into the house, the joy that a dog brings was back! Once again, I was complete. As my friend and my companion, despite having just met, I was a whole person again.

A little more than three years later, Andy's role as my pet hasn't changed. He brings me joy, happiness and fun every single day. It's hard not to laugh when you have a big smiling dog in front of you.

What has changed is that Andy also has a role in other people's lives as a therapy dog. With incredible breeding and consistent training, Andy is now able to enhance the lives of many more people. When we visit local hospitals, staff and visitors alike stop us countless times as we make our way through the hospital. People crouch down, giving him a hug and a pat, looking into his beautiful eyes. They tell him how he has just made their difficult day so much happier. Patients who are unable to speak and unable to move from their beds light up when they see Andy walk into their rooms. Situating himself next to them, he offers comfort by his mere presence.

As a therapy dog, Andy visits residents in nursing homes and walks with them as they wheel their chairs into the hallways. Often struggling to lean over and extend their hands, they pet his head and touch his back, reminding them of pets they have loved and miss so much.

One by one, Andy sits down next to them, gently resting his head on their knees. Patiently, he allows all who are in need to pet him.

As a reading companion, another form of pet therapy, Andy visits the libraries and listens while children read their favorite stories to him. Whether they are new readers or more experienced, Andy sits calmly as each child enjoys that loving experience of time spent with a very special dog.

I had no idea when I bought home this delicious puppy in the middle of winter that he would really be a loving companion for anyone but me. It's not anything I could have ever planned. But now, several years later, I am so fortunate to be able to share this amazing dog and let others experience the love and affection that I get to enjoy every single day.

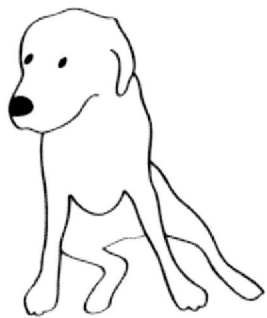

The Road to Pet Therapy

M any dog owners don't ever see their dogs as adults. Regardless of their age, they are, to us, puppies.

Andy has actually matured over the last three plus years. Most of the dish towel stealing has stopped and Andy pretty much walks right past my tee shirt lying on the floor without grabbing it. Never a big barker, he has always been a relaxed dog who wasn't bothered by noises or odd sounds. From early puppyhood, unless a dog was encroaching upon his territory, Andy was content.

Andy started working as a therapy dog when he was around six months old. Visiting my Dad in the hospital, Andy easily navigated through the equipment and was able to sit calmly next to the hospital bed so he could be petted.

Those hospital visits convinced me that Andy could be a great therapy dog candidate. He was certainly a confident dog. Even at his young age, he already knew basic obedience skills and was responsive when he was learning new things. Gentle and patient, Andy seemed to have the perfect temperament for therapy work.

He *was* young, though. Most therapy dogs usually don't begin their work until they are three or four years old. I needed to join a therapy group to show me the ropes and was fortunate enough to find a pet therapy group that welcomed young dogs.

After submitting a few membership and health documents, Andy and I joined the ranks of pet therapy volunteers.

It was a great indoctrination for me and for Andy. Visiting hospitals and nursing facilities, I was able to "get my feet wet" in the therapy world and assess my comfort level in these challenging environments. Even more importantly, the facilities enabled me to evaluate Andy's progress. And whether Andy, as such a young dog, could adapt and function in new places with minimal stress and anxiety.

Andy was a natural! He was amazingly tolerant and unfazed by the newness of an unknown facility. It was thrilling to see the happiness in whomever we encountered and the joy that was felt by anyone who petted Andy.

Feeling more comfortable and confident with my pet therapy work, I broke from the group and decided to try it on my own. I had great familiarity with a hospital near my home and had made friends at a nursing facility we had visited while a member of the original therapy group. It was wonderful to be able to take Andy on a whim and visit without the restriction of a schedule.

After almost two years of various pet therapy visits, I decided to pursue official pet therapy registration with a nationally recognized registry. As a registered dog, my opportunities for pet therapy would broaden and Andy could virtually give service in any pet therapy capacity in any facility.

In December of 2009, under the guidance and direction of Therapy Dogs, Incorporated, (TD, Inc.) I continued the pet therapy training. Although we were already quite experienced, over the course of the next few months, Andy and I visited all over town. Shops, restaurants, grocery stores - anywhere that welcomed a therapy dog in training. My goal was to expose Andy to as many people as possible and enable him to become comfortable with new and different situations. Andy and I had become a familiar sight in our "regular haunts" that even now, long after the training, when I go somewhere without him, people ask me where he is!

Andy and I were evaluated on four occasions by TD, Inc. testers, assessing our suitability as a pet therapy team. Happily, in early March of 2010, we passed all of the evaluations and became registered as an official pet-handler therapy team.

Today, as a registered therapy dog, Andy continues his hospital and nursing home work but has added a new role as a Canine Reading Companion. He is the "reading dog" at the Huntington Woods Public Library. We visit each week and Andy is available to children – and adults – who stop by to read, chat or just give him a quick pet.

As a reading companion, his job is twofold. Reading aloud to a dog enables children at all reading levels to enhance their enjoyment of reading while improving their literacy skills. As a member of the nationally recognized Canine Reading Education Assistance Dogs program, R.E.A.D., Andy gives children the opportunity to read in a non-judgmental manner, increasing their self-confidence and self-esteem. Secondly, as a reading companion, Andy helps children learn more about animals and how animals can have more of a role in our lives than simply being our loving pets.

Andy is a perfect therapy dog. He always knows when his vest goes on that his role is as a therapy dog, offering emotional comfort and affection to others.

For me, as his handler and owner, giving service with my dog adds an incredible dimension to my life that I didn't even know was missing. My world has been enlarged beyond measure and each new therapy visit continues to be gratifying and exciting. Although my experiences differ from one visit to another and the stories I recount involve different settings with different people, my reactions to the visits are quite the same. Therapy visits are happy joy filled moments that always impact someone in some way.

A dog's ability to provide therapy to others has nothing to do with age. Despite now being an adult dog and having some great experiences and credentials behind him, Andy is still my little blonde puppy. He will always be that to me.

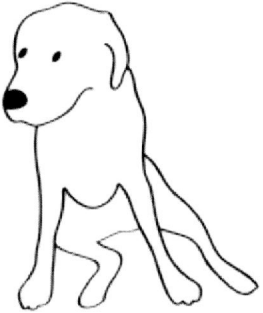

Andy Visits the Hospital

As the owner of a therapy dog, every new visit is a completely new experience despite having visited the facility many times. Some visits are more rewarding than others, some are more stressful for me and also for Andy. Regardless of whom we encounter, I know that the surprise of seeing a big yellow dog in the most unlikely place brings happiness to anyone who happens to see us.

It was a quiet Sunday afternoon when I decided to take Andy for a visit at a local hospital. A reunion, of sorts, since that is where his pet therapy career began.

Wearing comfy shoes and my hospital ID, with Andy suited up in his red therapy vest, we walked briskly into the hospital, through the security station and down the main corridor.

The first person we saw was an emergency room nurse. Apologizing for seeming pushy and insistent, she suggested that we visit her unit first, as she directed us through the large steel doors into her world.

We navigated through the equipment that lined the narrow halls into a sea of green curtains that divided the area. Makeshift hospital rooms were filled with stricken patients and worried families. A din filled the air as everyone nervously chatted, somehow trying to pass the time in this stress-filled, anxious place.

As I walked slowly with my canine companion, waiting family members peered out from their curtained enclaves, stunned to see a dog walking through the hallways. Saying my hellos, people felt comfortable asking if they could pet Andy. It was obvious that this wonderful animal had temporarily diverted their attention.

A patient that could not speak motioned for me to bring Andy to his bedside so he could pet him. A woman on a gurney, in tremendous pain and distress, turned and extended her hand to touch Andy's soft ears before being wheeled to her spot. And a little boy and girl, no more than five or six, called out in delight as we walked past their mother's room. Impulsively, they rushed out to hug Andy and laughed when he kissed them.

Like so many, I have also waited in these curtained cubicles. Worrying. Hoping. That is why this visit was such a special visit for me. I knew exactly what these people were experiencing.

Therapy, healing and the incredible impact that a dog can make. For a few minutes on a lazy Sunday, simply by sharing my dog, people could feel love and not fear.

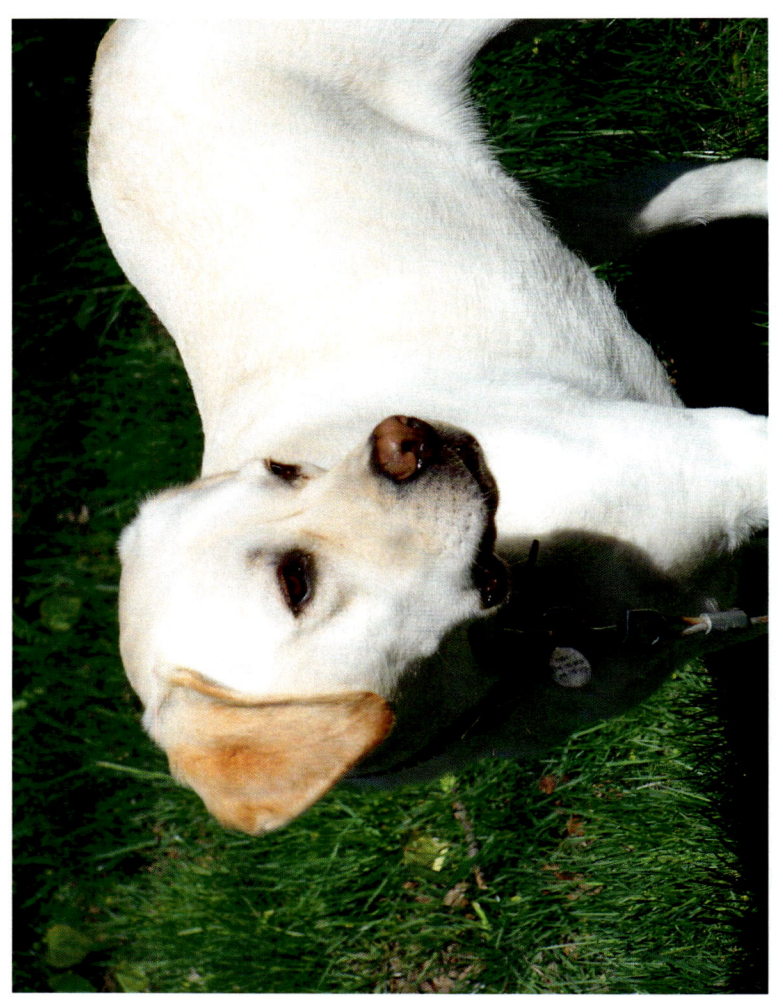

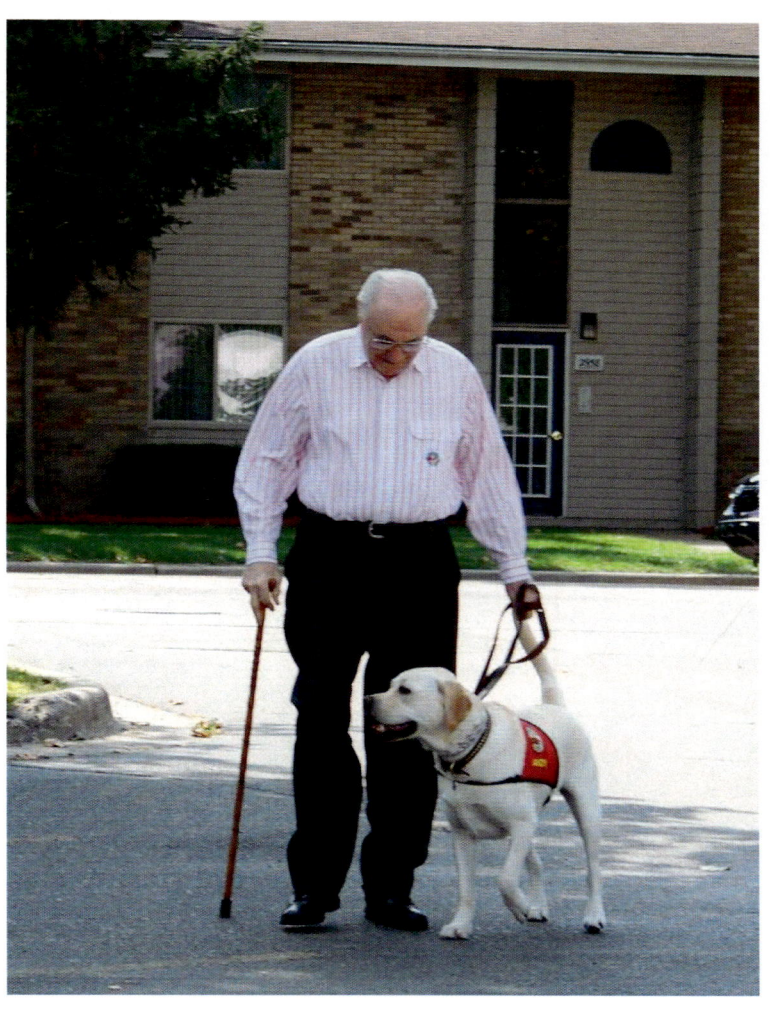

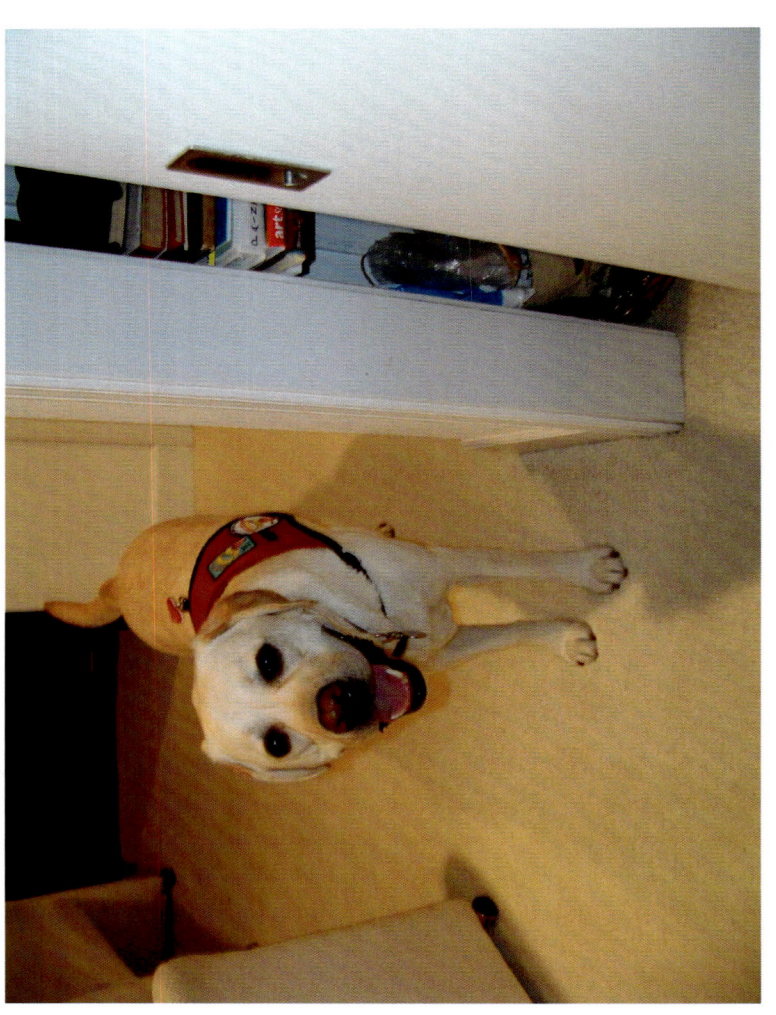

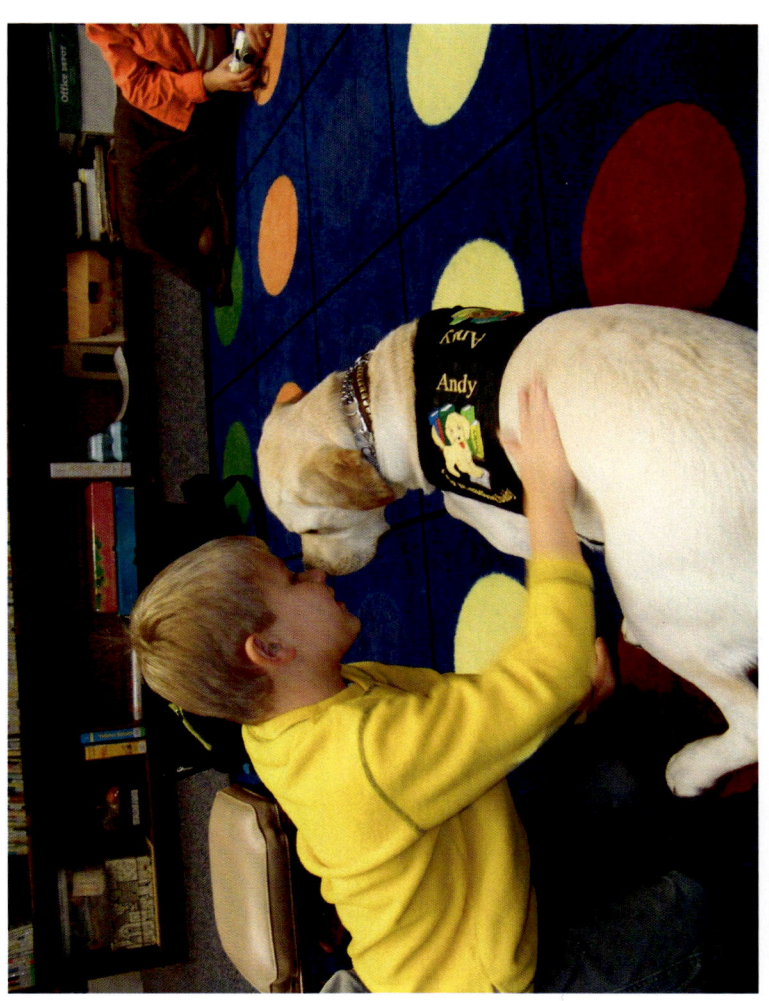

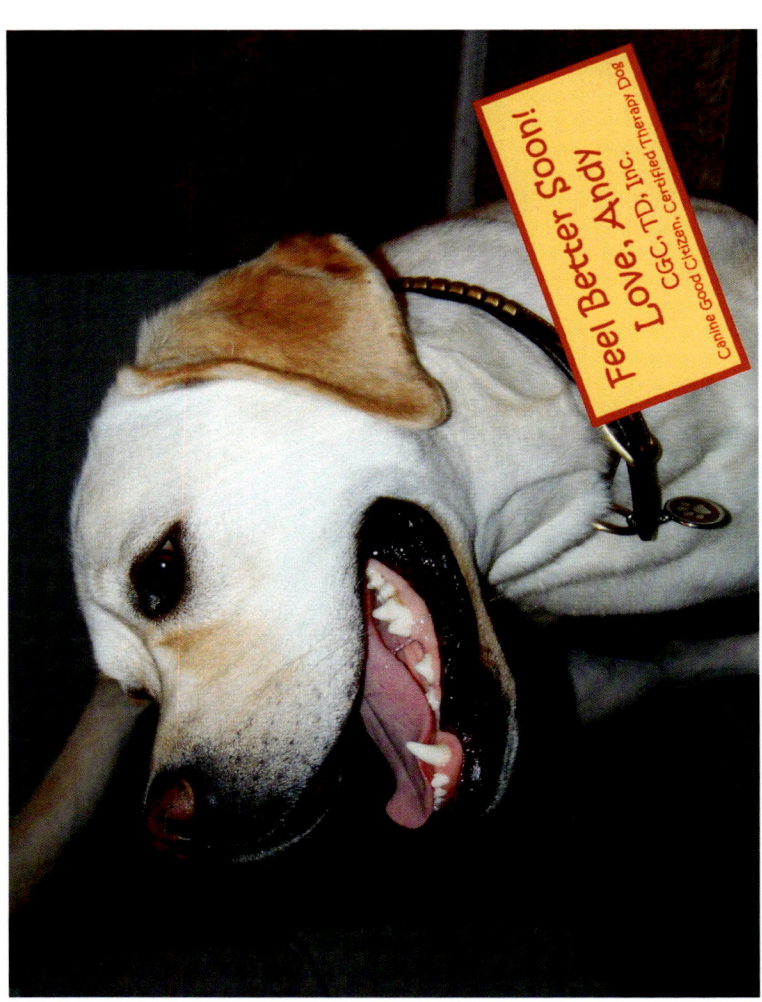

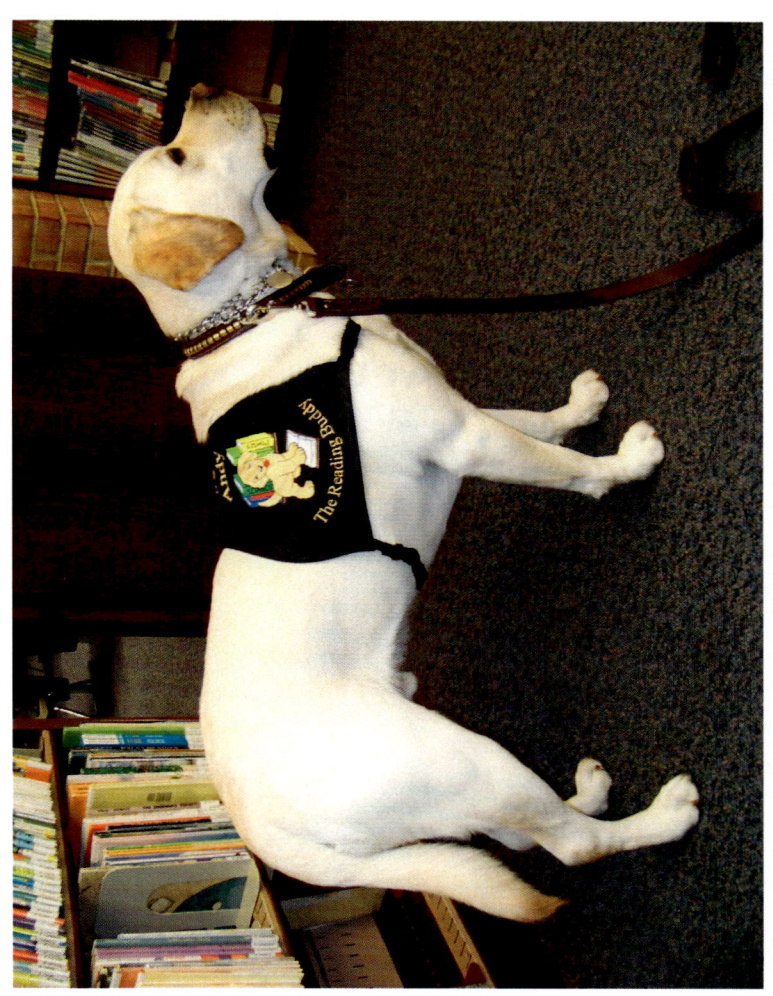

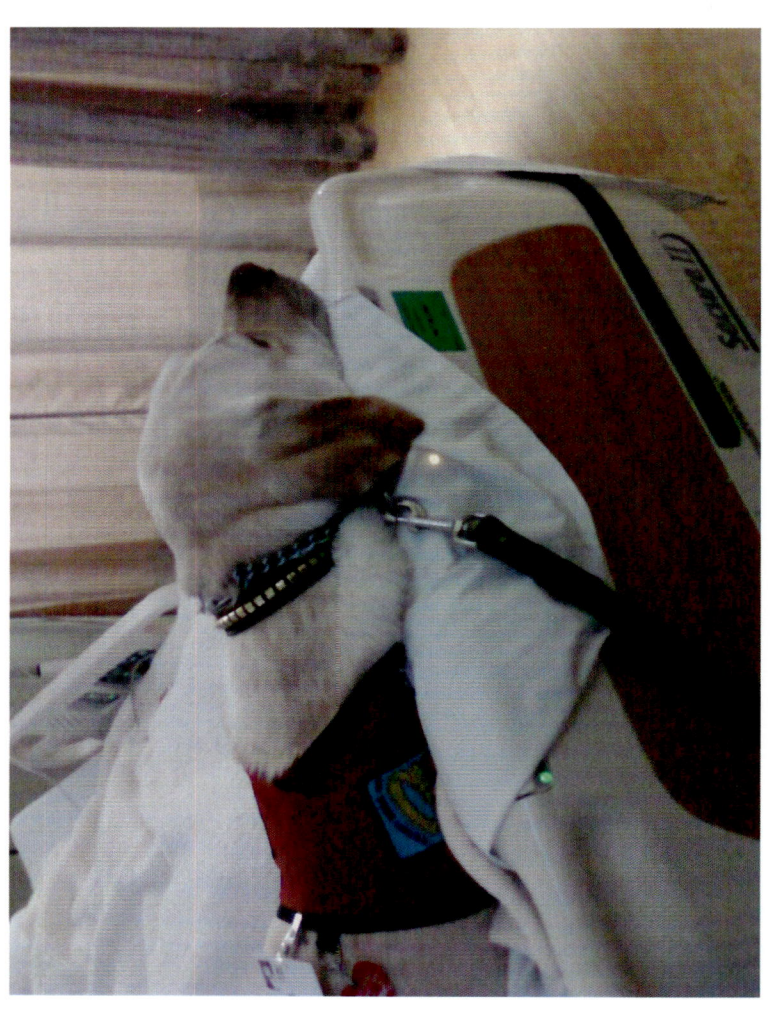

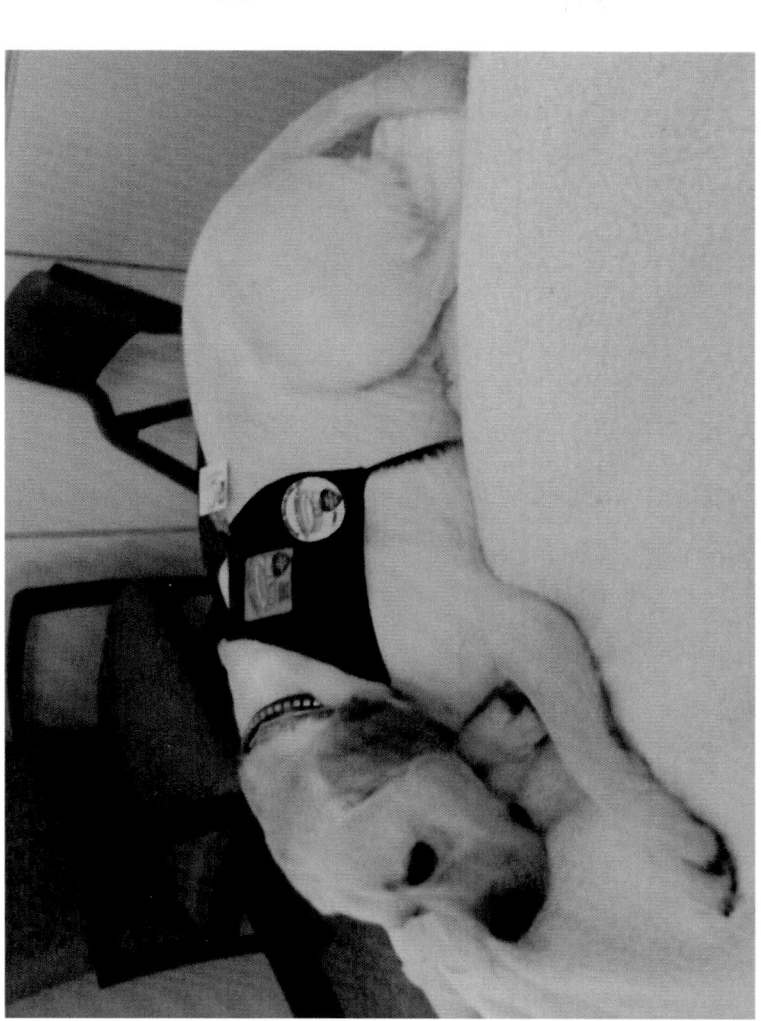

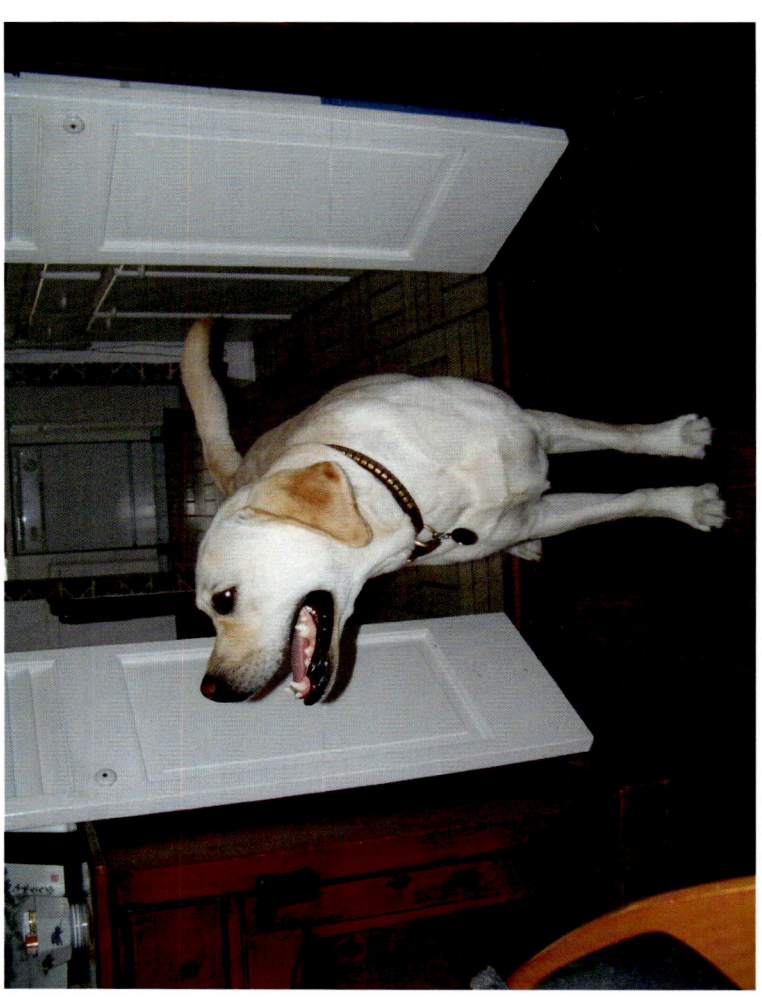

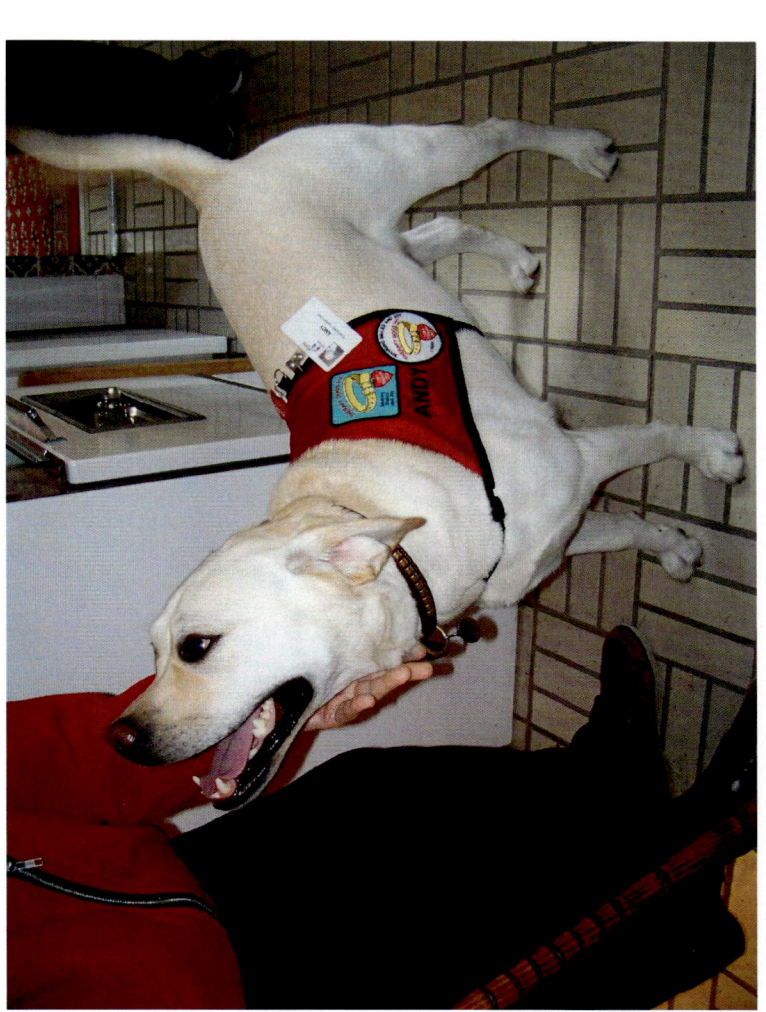

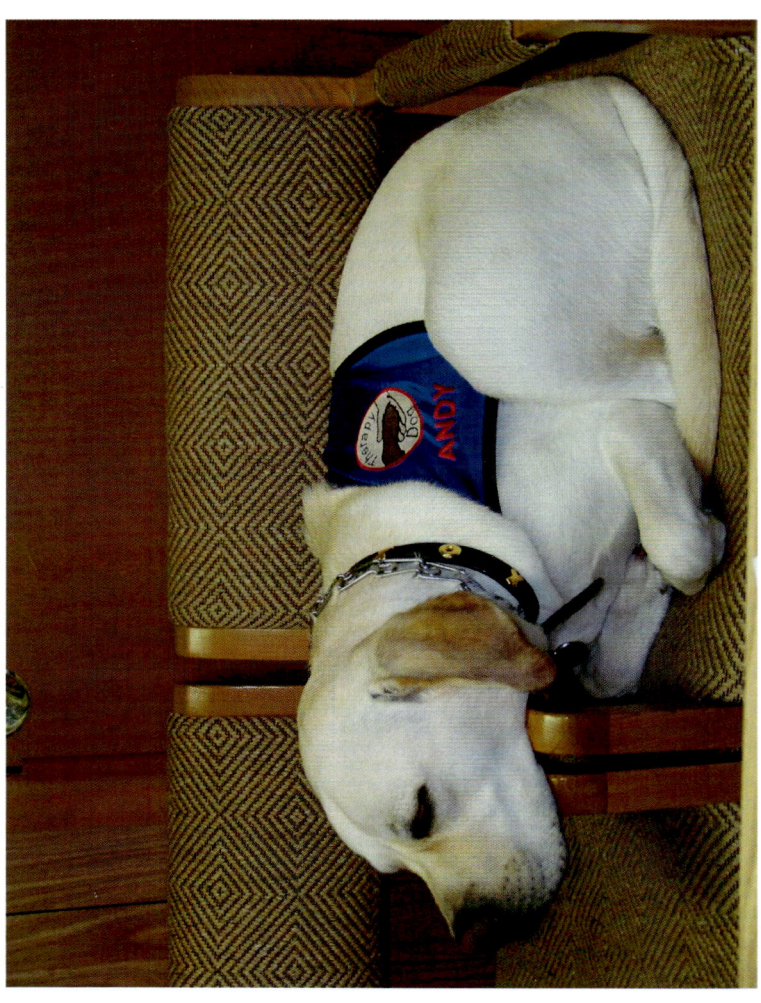

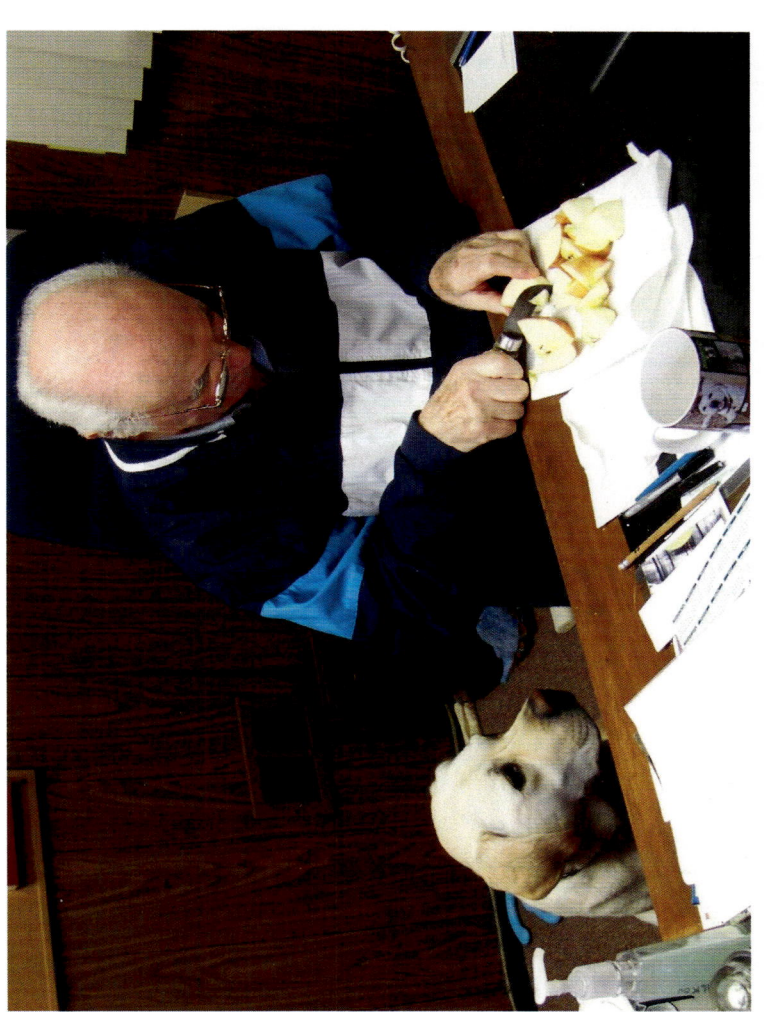

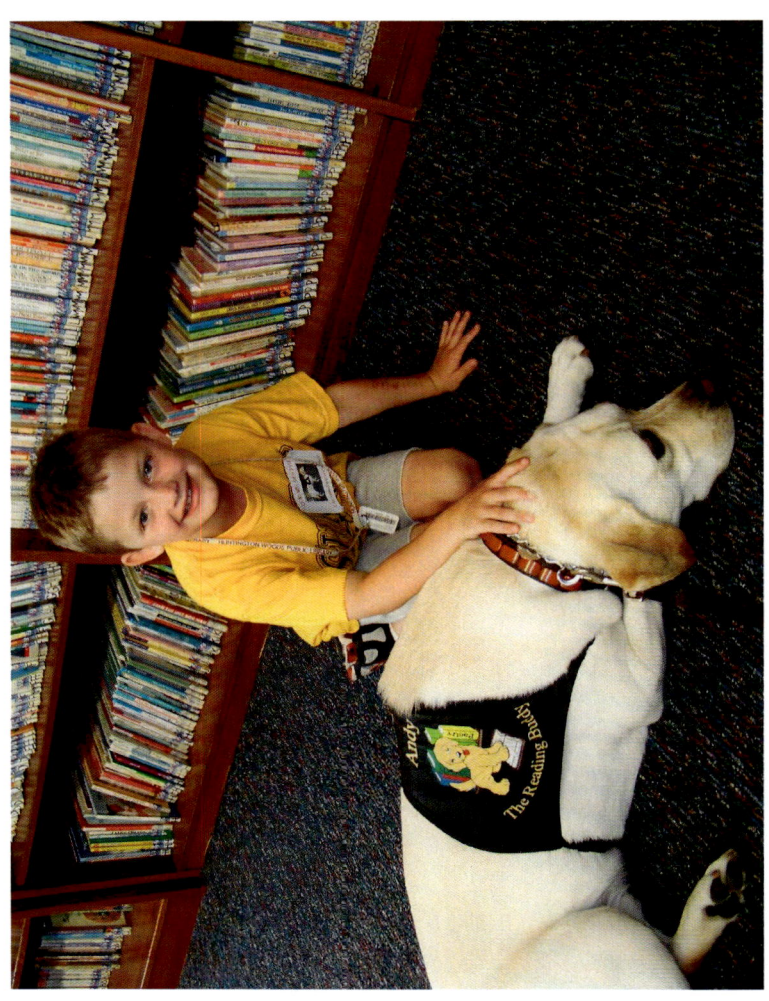

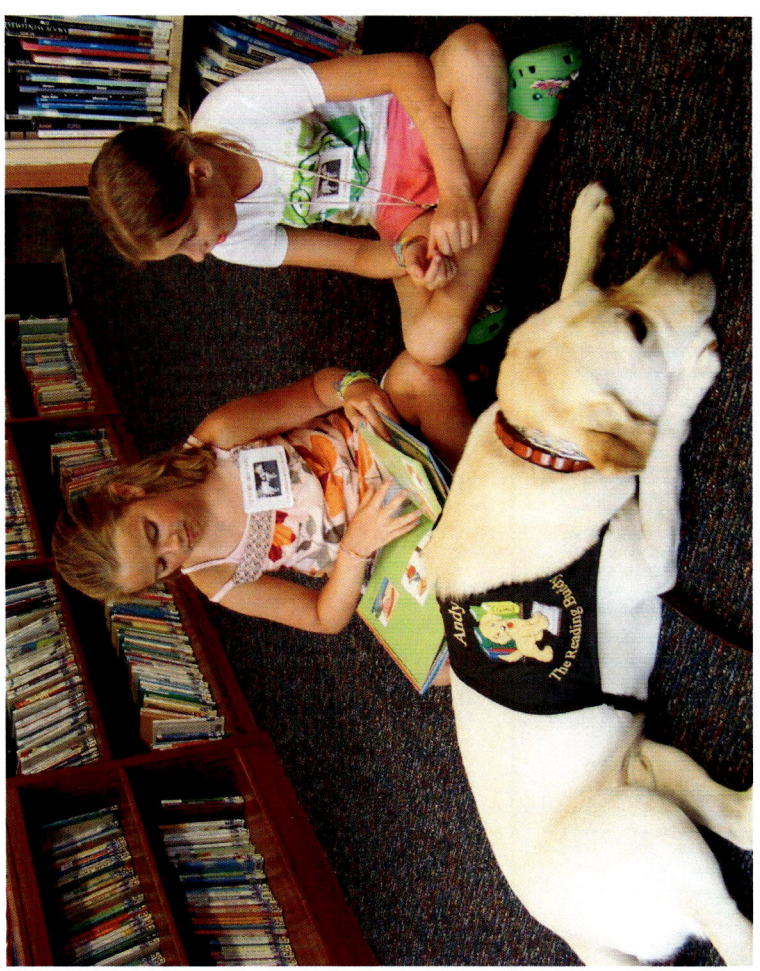

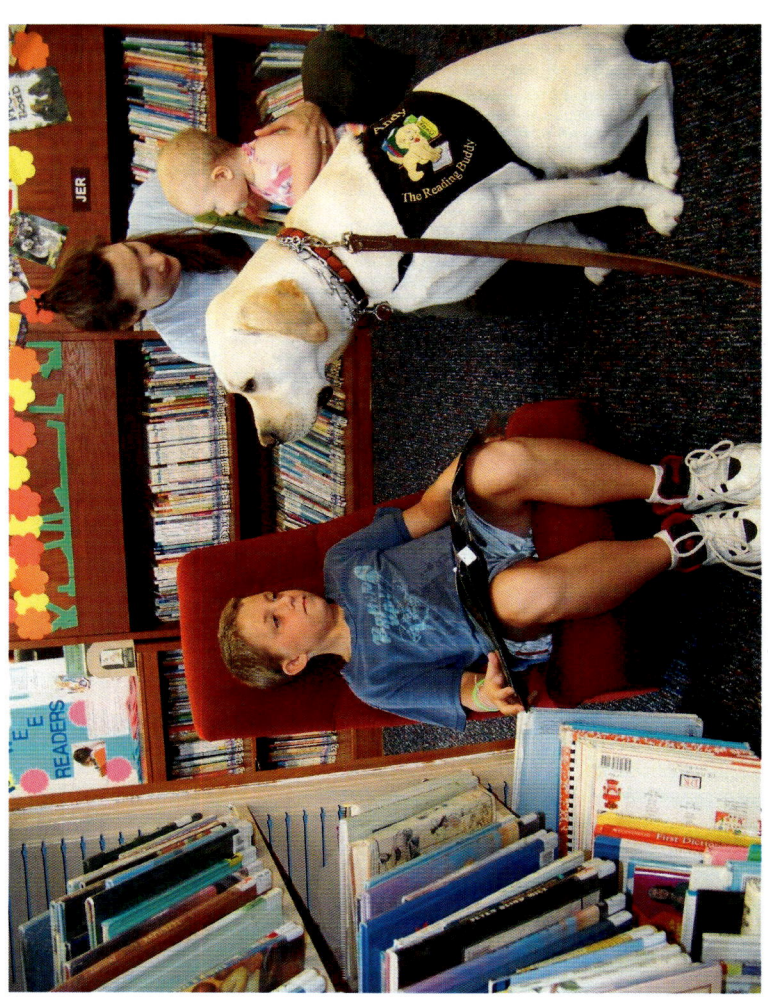

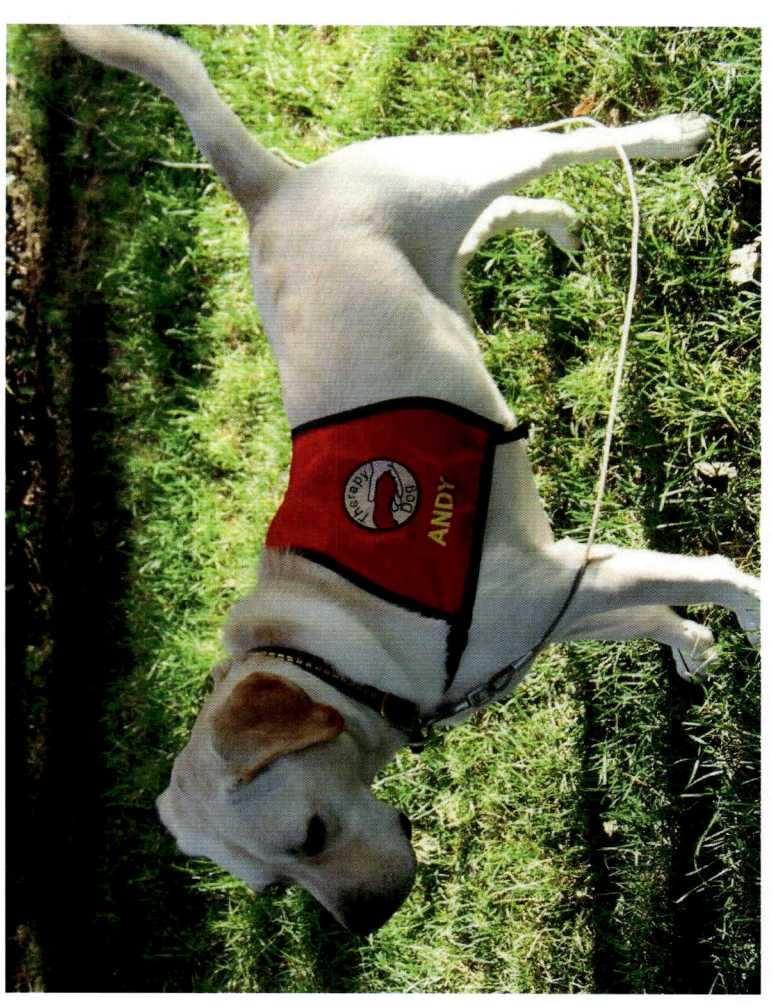

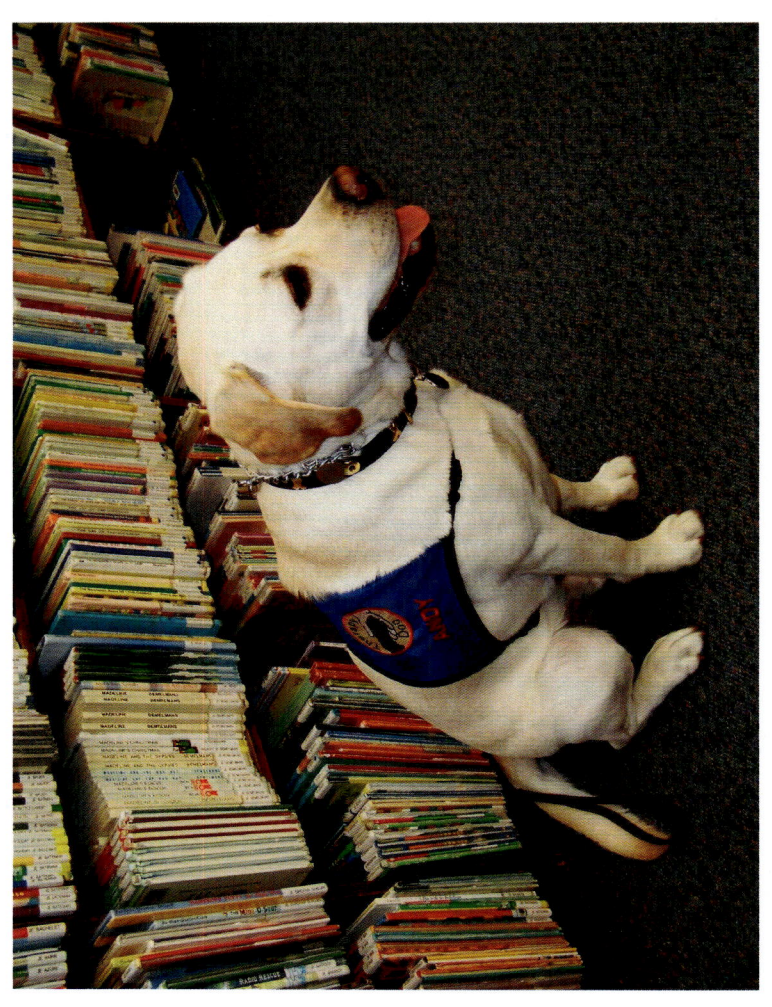

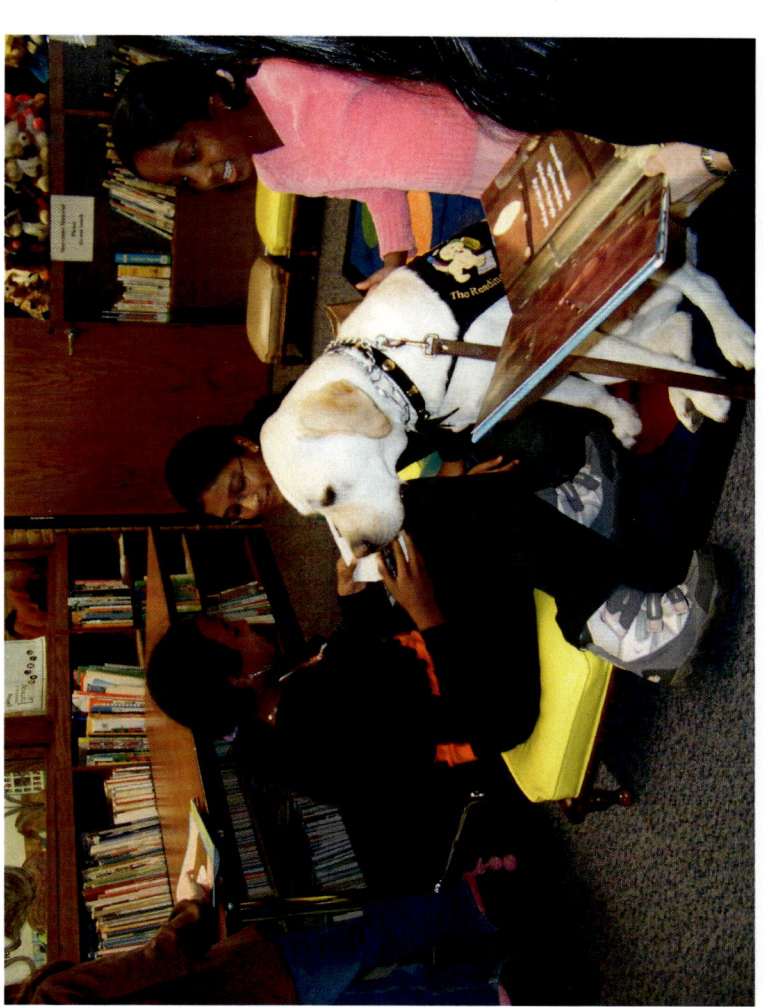

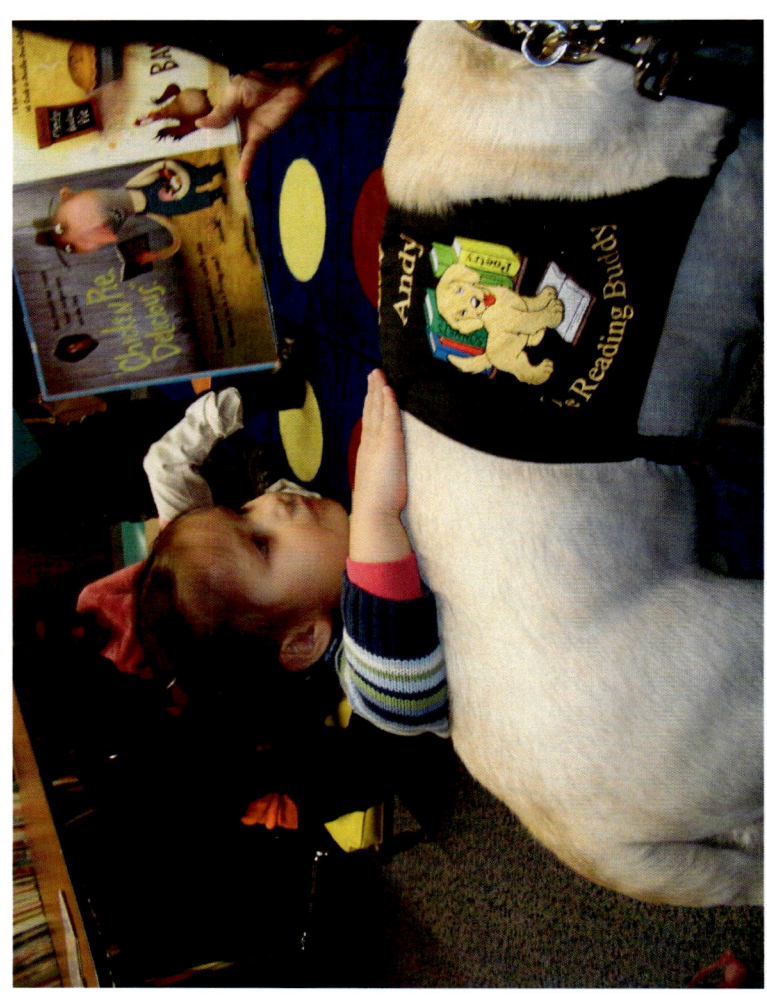

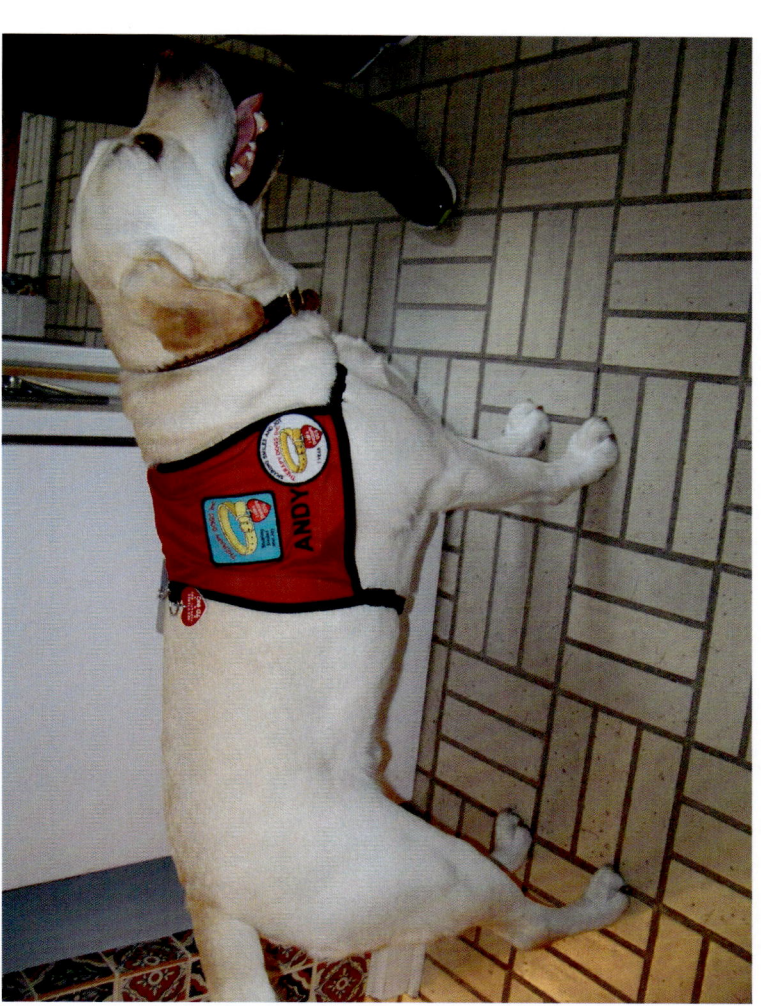

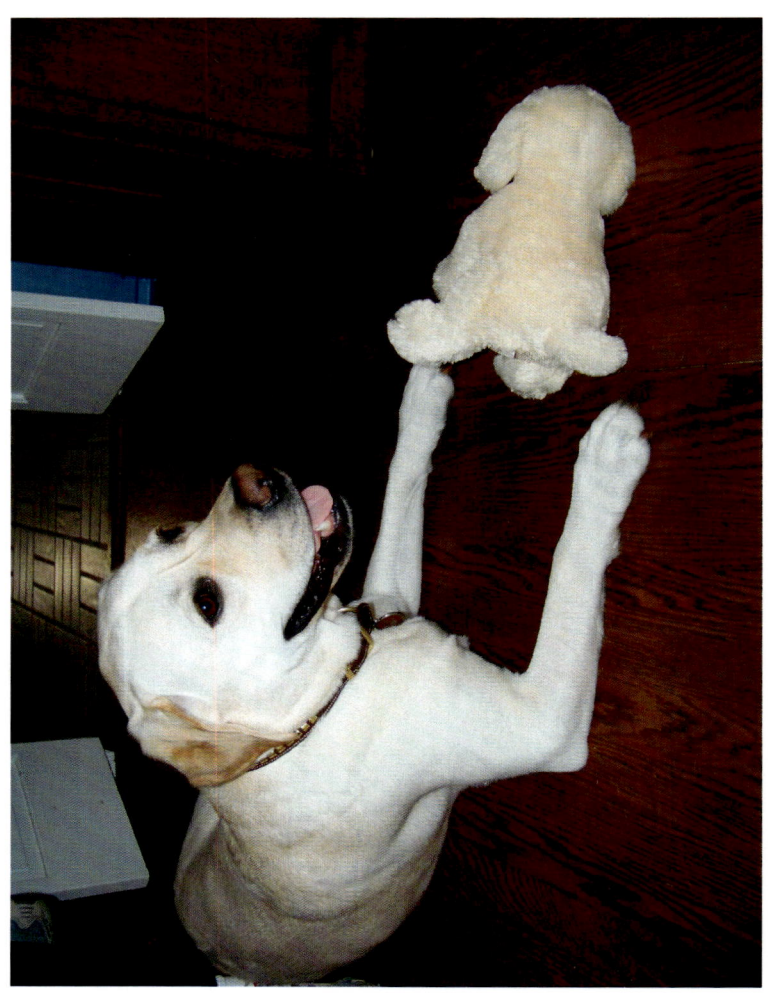

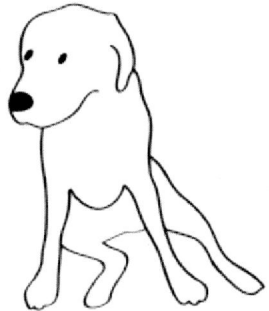

Keisha and Andy in The Space Room

Walking into the library with a dog is definitely not an everyday sight. Little kids will point, adults smile and a few dog lovers can't refrain from hugging Andy, unwilling to let him go.

Andy and I walked to our destination, The Space Room. An unusual room in the library that resembles the interior of a spaceship. It has colored lights, star-filled windows, and an astronaut floating above our heads. Lines of anxious children clamored about, getting ready to check-in for their reserved "Andy" reading time.

As a therapy dog and a canine reading companion, Andy listens to special stories that children choose just for him. It is the most incredible opportunity for a child to have a one-on-one experience in this super cool room with a sweet, cuddly and patient dog. It is their private reading time, where they won't be interrupted, corrected or criticized. A time where, for many kids, they do not have to compete for attention. It is, quite amazingly, a way that children at any level of proficiency can improve their reading skills and become comfortable reading out loud without feeling self-conscious or judged.

Most of the kids are pretty fearless. While many are literally eye-to-eye, or even in some cases, eye-to-nose with Andy, they pet him rather matter-of-factly, as if they have always seen a dog at the library.

Sometimes there is a child who apprehensively walks into the room, desperately wanting to read to Andy, but petrified of him at the same time. These are usually the same kids whose nervous parent exclaims, "Oh! He's a *real* dog! I thought he was a stuffed animal that sat next to the kids while they read!"

As six-year-old Keisha walked into The Space Room, I greeted her with smiles and a big Andy sticker for her tee shirt. Holding Andy's leash, I introduced her to him as he stood calmly next to me. As she clutched her mother's leg, I explained to Keisha that she could sit anywhere she wanted while she read. Even on her mother's lap, if she felt more comfortable.

A big part of my role in a pet therapy visit is to be very calm and put everyone at ease. I always give a little bit of information about the role of therapy animals and explain that Andy is a friendly, non-aggressive dog who has been specially trained. I tell both the children and their parents that Andy has terrific hearing and loves to listen to their stories, whether they are sitting on the floor next to him or reading to him from across the room.

With "Andy" stickers, bookmarks and embossed colorful "Reading with Andy" bracelets, I add to the experience. My goal is to make "Reading with Andy" a fun and memorable event. It is my hope that when the child's reading time with Andy has concluded, they will have enjoyed sharing their story with a dog and will have gained a better understanding of how animals can help people to improve their lives.

Keisha's reading selection was a book about a dog that goes camping. Despite her initial fears, she sat surprisingly close to Andy on a colorful cushion. Although she was trying to read her story, she could not avert her eyes from him as he lay nearby. Keisha was tempted to pet him but not quite sure how she should go about it.

As she continued her story, mostly turning the pages, she paused and asked me if Andy's fur was soft. In her barely audible voice, she asked how old he was, what he ate and what time he went to bed. Keisha was visibly intrigued.

Putting her fears aside, Keisha decided she *had* to pet him. With her timid outstretched hand, I held his head and instructed her to pet his tail and his back first. "That's an easy spot to pet him," I said. "Not too much going on there." Keisha pet Andy with resounding success.

Flashing her beaming, toothless smile, she decided she could do more. As I continued to hold Andy's leash, I told Keisha to ask Andy to sit down so she could pet his neck and the back of his head.

Thrilled that he had listened to her command, she pet Andy's head and ears and then, abandoning all fear, leaned down to give him a hug. Andy gave her a quick kiss and she giggled with .delight. Keisha's mother, watching her daughter overcome her enormous fear, was so overwhelmed that tears welled up in her eyes.

I am always amazed at the experiences I have when I am with Andy. Patient and attentive,

Andy's calm and gentle temperament allowed a child to overcome her fear. For Keisha and her mother, a huge breakthrough, hopefully, in discovering that animals can be enjoyed rather than feared.

As they exited The Space Room, Keisha turned back, thanked me and hugged Andy one last time and said, "See you next week, Andy!"

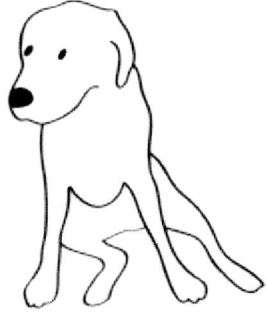

Saturday Mornings

Andy and I have been regular Saturday morning visitors at a local convalescent home for over a year. Some of the residents are temporary, arriving after a hospital stay for rehabilitation from surgery or to continue their recovery from less serious medical conditions. This is the interim stop before finally going back home.

Others, most that Andy and I see weekly, are long-term residents with permanent rooms. Their rooms represent an efficient consolidation of their personal belongings. Family photos hang on the walls, pretty objects dot the furniture and lace doilies transform this impersonal space into home. For most, this new home is the result of a serious life-changing illness or the inability to live as independently as they once did.

As we have become part of the regular weekend scenery, I have a familiarity not only with the staff but also many of the residents. Although we rarely introduce ourselves or refer to each other by name, we greet each other like old friends, as if we have been acquainted for years.

The appearance of a person walking a dog through the halls is glaringly noticeable. Wheelchair-bound residents line the corridors and common areas, watching as Andy and I walk slowly around the facility.

They wave and shout hellos, hoping we will make them our first stop.

Andy offers himself to each person, knowing instinctively that he must be gentle and patient. Many residents are able to hold onto Andy's strong paws quite easily, despite their often frail conditions, and pet his head and neck with vigor.

The joy he brings to them is immediately apparent. Andy uplifts their spirits and manages, in just a few short moments, to infuse them with energy and happiness.

As they pet Andy, we chat. I tell them a little bit about myself and about Andy. And as we visit, they have the opportunity to share a story and reminisce about their life with someone new who is interested and eager to listen.

The most common story I hear is that for many residents, the biggest adjustment they must make is living with the absence of their pets. I am certain this issue is rarely discussed, especially when the concern among family members is getting their relative settled.

As an independent and healthy person, bringing my dog, Andy, into this animal-free environment is a small way that I can ease that transition for others. Pet therapy visits help me make life for many residents a little more like it had always been.

I am asked many times if visiting a nursing facility is upsetting or emotionally difficult. Although I am frequently the only visitor many residents may have, I rarely feel discomfort or distress. I am always aware that my goal with pet therapy is to walk into a facility with a smile, bring a light-hearted attitude and share my beautiful dog.

Giving and sharing joy is the pleasure of pet therapy. With my loving dog standing next to me, leading the way forward, it is my passion, my avocation. That is the true reward of sharing kindness with someone else.

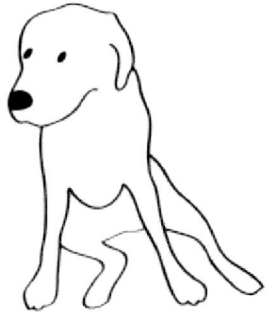

The Ho-Hum ER

Some days, the pet therapy visits to the emergency room are kind of ho-hum. That sounds kind of funny considering that everyone is there for some kind of emergency or another. Even though I'm not always in the mood, my weekly visits are a commitment I have with myself. To take an hour or two and share my remarkable dog. Hopefully, making a difference for someone else.

Andy and I went from one treatment area to another on one rather un-busy Sunday. I was struck by how many vacant rooms there were. A good thing, but definitely weird compared to the hustle-bustle that is the ER norm.

Although there were a few visits and certainly a few smiles along the way, it was not one of my more noteworthy experiences. It felt almost – *almost* – like just clocking in some time.

As we walked down a deserted corridor, I suddenly had one of those "light bulb" moments. This was not about making *me* feel better or gaining recognition for having shared my dog. The whole purpose of pet therapy – and what I reminded myself of – was about bringing some joy and happiness to someone *else's* day. My own satisfaction with sharing my dog was a bonus.

With this visit, even in the "ho-hum-ness" of the ER, someone enjoyed my loving dog. Someone got to feel that momentary diversion from their emergency and enjoy friendship and kindness in the most unconditional way.

Every visit does make a difference. Every visit touches someone. My goal with pet therapy is that I am a conduit toward that end.

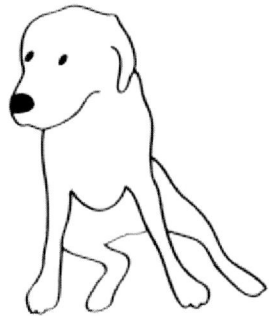

About Harold

Each visit to a hospital or nursing home is all about bringing good cheer and sharing a lighter moment at a time that is usually stressful. Walking in with a big yellow dog immediately affects the mood in a positive way.

In a hospital, especially, people are usually there

unexpectedly. They have had little or no time to make preparations for even a little bit of comfort.

In a nursing facility, most of the population is made up of permanent residents. People whom, for one reason or another, find themselves in a new setting and most often, the place that will be their last home.

When I bring Andy for a therapy visit, I enter the facility smiling and upbeat. Our visits are happy experiences. A wonderful distraction from the sameness of the day. Visits allow me to relate some amusing therapy experiences, talk about current events and give people the opportunity to enjoy my fabulous dog.

With few exceptions, I have no personal relationship with most of the people that we visit. I am able to move through a facility without experiencing too much distress or upset. Although I certainly feel compassion for the people we visit, there is an emotional detachment that enables me to function in these environments.

I suppose that is how doctors and nurses function as well. Compassionate, but detached.

In recent months, I took Andy to visit a dear family friend. A lovely, sweet man named Harold. He had been in and out of the hospital and in and out of the nursing facility many times. Despite not being the same energetic man I had always known, Harold was always ready to receive a fun visit from Andy and me. He was so grateful and appreciative that I took the time to bring Andy to see him.

It was as much therapy for me as it was for him. Harold was a fantastic storyteller. During these visits I could enjoy more of his terrific stories, hear the latest about his kids and bring him up to date on the comings and goings with my family.

Visits with Harold had an emotional component, of course, because this was a man whom I had known for over forty years. Hardly just another man down the hall - this was a friend that I loved.

Harold passed away this week. A most incredible

man with a loving family and a wealth of friends. A man that made an impact on everyone that knew him. He had a special feeling for all of his friends. And made them all feel as special as he was.

It is always a privilege to share my dog with people. When Andy looks up at someone with his kind and loving eyes, it's hard not to experience his love.

I hope Harold felt that. I know he enjoyed our visits. I hope he knew that not only was I there to share the sweetness of my dog, but friendship and love from someone whose life he surely touched.

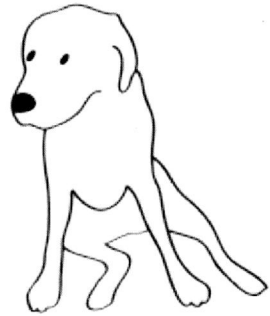

The Library Dog is Mr. Boy

I really do feel like the Pied Piper when I walk into the library with Andy. Eyes turn and people look on in shock that I am brazenly walking a dog into a library. Kids usually begin whispering to each other, "I didn't know you could bring a dog into the Library?"

As Andy and I walked in at our appointed time

last Thursday, the bevy of little girls waiting exclaimed, "There's Andy!" It is truly the most wonderful greeting anyone could imagine. No less than five girls, ages six to seven, swarmed Andy. They hugged and pet him and told Andy how much they missed him. It was adorable.

After scrambling to grab some suitable books, the girls formed their own line to take turns reading their stories. Some kids are shy at first, not really believing that a dog will want to hear them read. Some are a little fearful to get so close to Andy. But most are just thrilled that they get to pet him while they read. And, if they situate themselves just right, Andy will plop down right on their feet.

Today's stories were mostly dog stories. Although Andy occasionally gets to hear about the latest sports car or scientific discovery, for the most part, the kids who read to him chose stories about animals. Story after story, Andy patiently listened to everyone, allowing all of the petting and cuddling that came his way.

After the third or fourth story, one little girl, who hadn't yet chosen her book, urgently dashed off in pursuit of the perfect story to read. When she returned, she was holding a small square book. There was a photograph of a Labrador retriever puppy on the front cover. She came over to me and whispered, "I thought Andy would love this book. Look at this cute dog. It looks just like him!" she said.

I smiled and quietly told her that as soon as her friend had finished reading, I would share a great story about the book she had just chosen.

As the last word was read, the crowd of kids all asked, "What are you going to tell us?"

With all eyes upon me, I said, "That little book about the dog that your friend just picked? That is a book that *I* wrote. That book *is* all about Andy."

They were stunned! They eagerly flipped through the pages, exclaiming how Andy had grown as they compared him to his cute puppy pictures.

For the kids? True astonishment that they actually *knew* the dog in a library book *and* the author that wrote the book.

For me? Seeing the thrill of the kids as they discovered Andy's puppy past was the most unexpected joyful moment.

Sharing experiences with these great kids, I'm sure they would agree ... there is little doubt that a dog makes everything more fun!

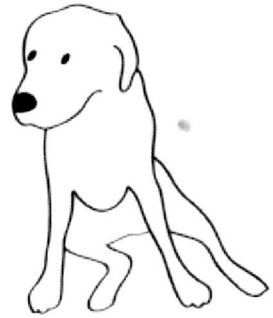

The Familiar Comfort of a Dog

When I decided to train Andy as a therapy dog, it really was because he was at ease in so many situations. That, combined with his loving and gentle nature, seemed to be the perfect combination for therapy work. I loved the idea of having a dog that would be welcomed into a variety of places.

A dog that was so well-received his presence alone would bring joy and comfort to anyone who came in contact with him.

Having a therapy dog is all about helping others. Many people have said that simply glancing at Andy from across the room or giving him a quick pat on his head provided comfort and relief to them in some manner. If there were no other remarkable experiences, it would still be abundantly clear that providing comfort to others was why I trained my dog, Andy, as a therapy dog.

Today, however, was a pet therapy experience that struck deep to the core. A realization why humans and animals are so valuable to each other. Each incredible species offers comfort and unconditional friendship to the other. For a moment, for an instant, that can impact a lifetime.

I was at the hospital with Andy visiting my Mom, who was a patient awaiting surgery. He sat with her on the bed, enjoying all the cuddles and hugs she gives him in her "regular" life.

When we left her room, as is always the case with a pet therapy visit, leaving the floor and actually making our way out of the building takes a while. There is no such thing as a quick getaway with a dog.

Andy is a most tolerant and patient boy. He allows anyone who crosses his path to get their dose of therapy in their hectic day. Patients or staff, the result is the same. Smiles, happiness, calm. Whatever their day had been about was now about seeing a beautiful dog.

As Andy and I walked to leave the floor, a nurse approached me. She explained she had a patient that was huge dog lover and her family was unable to arrange a visit from her own dogs. The nurse asked that we visit her patient and pointed out the direction to her room. We were on the way!

As we approached the room, there was a lot of commotion outside. Family members, doctors, other hospital staff bustled about. In the crowd, a man wearing a firefighter's tee shirt asked if he could pet Andy. He mentioned that his mother had been a breeder of Labrador retriever dogs for over fifty years. Pointing into the room, he asked if we could stop inside, not knowing that visiting his mother was already our mission. The firefighter told me she was gravely ill and could not speak at all. In all likelihood, she would offer little recognition of Andy. The commotion outside of her room was the hospital staff in consultation, making the arrangements for her final days in hospice care.

She was, in fact, dying.

With Andy's red leash firmly in my grip, we walked in. I was smiling and cheery as Andy led the way around all of the tubes and beeping machines. The firefighter's mother could clearly see us but lay still. I introduced her to Andy and told her a little bit about him. I explained that he was a registered therapy dog who especially loved to visit dog lovers.

Andy carefully inched his way to her bedside and looked at her, placing his head as closely as possible to her frail hand.

And there it was. A glimmer of recognition. A little sparkle in her eyes as she saw this big yellow dog at her side. I lifted Andy's front paws onto her bed so she could reach them more easily. Holding some dog treats in my closed hand, I placed my hand next to hers and Andy licked her fingers.

With her family watching, trying to offer her some comfort in these difficult moments, she smiled. That cold wet nose and familiar dog kisses were what she had known for a lifetime.

It was, as it had always been for this family, a dog that could offer this fragile woman comfort and affection.

The power of a dog's love. Unconditional. Freely given. Without any regard for someone's circumstances or station in life.

Love that truly lasts a lifetime.

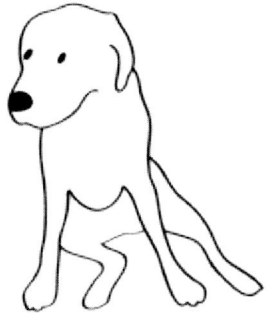

Making Me Laugh

The visits with the kids that come to the library are, without a doubt, completely fun and amusing therapy experiences. Putting aside the seriousness of pet therapy and the "Reading with Andy" program, the kids are simply delighted and thrilled at being able to hang out with a dog.

Most of the books the kids read have something to do with animals. Today however, almost everyone read from cookbooks. Preparing for a City-wide bake-off, the kids were pouring through recipes to find what they hoped would be the winning entry. Brownies, popcorn balls, petal-shaped pancakes, trail mix – everything sounded so delicious.

As Andy lay within petting distance of all of the kids, they took turns reading their selections. Every part of each recipe was read precisely and in exact detail. From the recommended pan to the proper oven temperature, by the time the last child had explained how to blend butter with chocolate, we were all licking our lips, including Andy!

As we continued around the circle, one little girl confessed she was a bad cook. She said she was, "*definitely* not entering the bake-off," but kept us laughing by reading a series of sports-related knock-knock jokes.

Sprinkled in between the recipes and the jokes, kids pointed out their latest bike injuries, told me all about their scooter mishaps and shared camp adventures. Almost apologetically, some kids even expressed that future family travel plans meant they would not be coming back to see Andy until the fall.

Today's library day was one of those truly wonderful visits where the party-like atmosphere was all because everyone just wanted to read to a dog.

We were all having such fun. By simply reading together, laughing and petting a dog, we all felt happy and relaxed.

This incredible exchange between humans and animals is the essence of the canine reading program. Today, it was canine pet therapy at its finest.

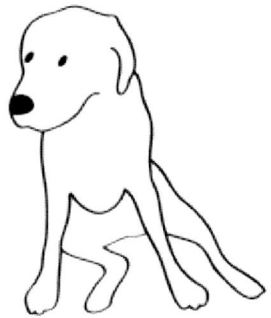

The Love of a Dog

How can you explain love? How can you possibly express why one day it isn't there and the next day it is? It's like trying to describe a flavor. You know it's delicious but you can't find the words that will truly convey it.

For many people, owning a dog just makes sense. As a service animal to a disabled person, as a watchdog to protect property or as a search and rescue dog for the military, it is simply a practical decision.

It may be coincidental that a dog has "landed" in your home and you agree you'll keep it. It is a decision in all likelihood, based on convenience and has nothing to do with emotion.

Whatever the reason, for many people, a dog may initially meet a very functional need.

For many of us, a dog is an extension of ourselves. It is what expands our ability to be unconditionally loving and giving. Through our dogs, we express kindness, generosity and can share the joy in our lives. We simply *need* a dog for our own existence.

In exchange for our dogs making us feel more complete, we undertake the responsibility of care. A seemingly minor tradeoff for something that gives us so much.

I have always had a need to explain things, to analyze why and how things exist. Maybe this time, for me, a consummate dog lover, the only thing I really need to explain is that my life is happier and more fulfilled when I have a dog. It might actually be that it is not so much about trying to explain love, but just accepting it.

I can do that.

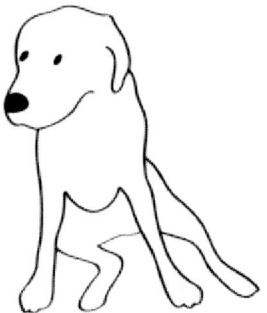

Our Therapy Dogs

Every day for almost two years, Andy has come to my office with me. He runs into the building, stops in front of my office door and waits for me to open up. Within a few minutes of my arrival, my Dad usually arrives. And so the fun for Andy - and my Dad - begins.

Each day, Andy sits patiently while my Dad prepares a specially cut apple for him. After the apple, Andy brings a huge bone to my Dad. Settling next to his chair, he'll chomp away on one end as my Dad holds onto the other. A quick game of fetch follows, then a little nap, with Andy finally situating himself once again right next to my Dad's chair. It is a wonderful time for Andy and a wonderful, loving time for my Dad. Both look forward to this daily ritual.

Although not every dog can walk into an office or a hospital or a library, every dog actually *is* a therapy dog. Simply by their presence in our lives, our dogs keep us emotionally grounded through their love and companionship.

They are the uncritical sounding boards for our ideas and the true, patient friends that tirelessly listen to our concerns and worries.

Dogs take us outside of ourselves and give us something else to think about and care for. They offer us love and comfort because that is the essence of what they are made of. They are the very definition of unconditional love and friendship.

Having a dog gives us focus and purpose to our

lives. Helping us to add order to our days, they help us to structure each day and provide routine.

They create memories for us – happy and sad – and they allow us to quiet the busyness of life.

The goal of pet therapy is to offer an animal to another person to provide affection and quite simply, to make them feel good. The pleasure and joy we receive from our own dogs is exactly that.

As the passionate owner of a remarkable dog, I can say with the utmost certainty that Andy absolutely provides that for me. Whether it is in his regular "dog life" or when he is working in a pet therapy capacity, through his contact with others, he provides that for them as well.

It is my hope that Andy and I will have a long therapy career ahead of us. But whether he continues to touch the lives of others or settles in to enjoy his wonderful life with me, I sure know of no better way to live.

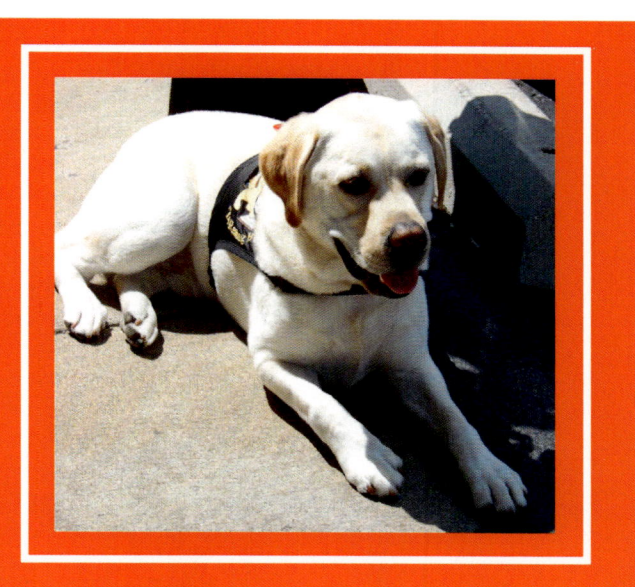

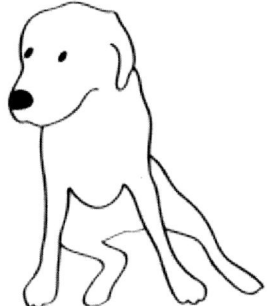

Goodbye.